Earth-Friendly Fitness

Sustainable Tips and Practices for Active Lifestyles

Table of Contents

Chapter 1. Introduction

Welcome to an inspiring journey towards a healthier you and a greener Earth! Our Special Report on 'Earth-Friendly Fitness: Sustainable Tips and Practices for Active Lifestyles,' stands as a beacon of motivation, guiding you towards a fitness regime that not only benefits your wellbeing but also harmonizes with our planet's health. Embark on a new era of fitness, where the sweat you shed contributes to a greener world, without compromising on your health and fitness objectives. From sustainable exercise routines, eco-friendly workout gear, to organic dietary habits, this enlightening report encapsulates it all! So fasten your eco-conscious fitness straps and prepare to dive into a realm where fitness meets sustainability. This report doesn't just aim to shape you, but also the future of our beautiful planet. A purchase promises infinite value - an investment not only in yourself but in the world we inhabit and cherish. Welcome aboard on your 'Earth-Friendly Fitness' journey!

Chapter 2. Understanding the Intersection of Fitness and Sustainability

To navigate our journey through sustainable fitness effectively, it's crucial to first understand the intersection between fitness and sustainability. The era of unconscious fitness routines is slowly receding, making way for a more conscientious approach, one that intertwines personal health and ecological health. This change is supported by the ever-increasing evidence of human activities impacting the ecosystem, leading many to rethink their approach towards health and exercise, factoring in the environmental dimensions.

2.1. A New Perspective

Think of fitness as a spectrum where one end signifies individual health, and the other represents the health of the environment. It's a delicate balancing act where an enhancement in one aspect should ideally not be detrimental to the other. But that unfortunately, is often not the case.

For instance, bottled water consumed in gyms is a significant source of plastic waste. Similarly, energy-intensive treadmills and cycles, other gym equipment manufactured and shipped from overseas, trendy but environmentally harmful clothing materials, promotion of non-organic supplements, and long-distance travel to workout locations all contribute to environmental stress. It's not to say we should abandon exercises or gyms, but rather, it's time we reviewed our choices and revised them to make responsible decisions.

2.2. Earth-Friendly Workout Regimes

One of the core aspects towards a sustainable and healthy lifestyle is choosing workout regimes that emphasize minimal environmental impact. Opt for activities that require less equipment or invest in equipment made from sustainable materials.

Outdoor activities like running, hiking, swimming, cycling, or yoga keep carbon footprints in check and can even offer therapeutic benefits of being in nature. Like the concept of 'Plogging' (picking up litter while jogging) which is steadily gaining momentum, altruistic fitness activities can double up to serve the environment.

2.3. Sustainable Gear and Apparel

Just as the fitness regime, the gear and apparel we choose play a significant role in sustainable fitness. Opting for eco-friendly gear made from recycled materials or sustainably harvested resources can greatly reduce the environmental damage associated with production and disposal of synthetic gear.

Companies are now offering workout apparel made with organic cotton, recycled polyester, and even unique materials like algae and bamboo. By supporting such businesses, you help foster an industry that's not damaging to the planet.

2.4. Organic and Locally Sourced Nutrition

The dietary choices we make as part of our fitness plan significantly influence sustainability. Encouraging a diet rich in organic, locally sourced produce reduces carbon emissions associated with transporting food from far-off places. Additionally, these foods are often more nutritious as they're harvested at peak ripeness and aren't subjected to artificial ripening or long storage times.

2.5. Energy-Effective Gyms

While most traditional gyms are energy-intensive due to their need for powered equipment, lighting, and climate control, a new breed of "green gyms" has emerged as an alternative. These gyms utilize energy-efficient equipment, utilize natural light, advocate minimized water use, and even produce their own energy through solar panels and workout machines that generate electricity.

2.6. Conscious Disposal and Recycling

Finally, the disposal of fitness gear, supplements, and food packaging contributes significantly to environmental degradation. Conscious choices about recycling, reusing, and composting can help mitigate this. We should opt for biodegradable or recyclable packaging, donate old workout gear for reuse, and compost organic waste whenever possible.

Understanding the intersection of fitness and sustainability is not just about rethinking our workout routines, eating habits, or gym choices. It's about adopting a holistic view of our lifestyle. It challenges us to question our habits, demands conscious decision-making, and promotes an awareness that extends from personal health to the health of our planet. The rewards for this shift are bountiful - a healthier you, a thriving environment, and the assurance of a sustainable future.

Chapter 3. The Rise of Green Gyms: Eco-friendly Workouts that Energize

In the fitness industry, green gyms have emerged as an innovative approach to exercise, marrying the pursuit for health and fitness with environmental responsibility. Embracing the ethos of sustainability, green gyms are revolutionizing our traditional exercise spaces and methods while empowering fitness enthusiasts to make more Earth-friendly choices.

3.1. Understanding Green Gyms

Green gyms, or eco-gyms, are fitness centers designed to minimize energy consumption and waste, while maximizing sustainability. These gyms are built from recycled materials and are often powered by renewable energy sources. They run on innovative, self-sustaining exercise equipment that generates electricity as users workout, transforming fitness routines into opportunities for energy production.

Indoor green gyms effectively reduce the carbon footprint associated with traditional gym settings. They utilize LED lighting, motion sensors, and other energy-efficient fittings. Additionally, they implement water-saving devices and incorporate recycled or sustainably sourced items for furnishings, from yoga mats to towels. All these factors contribute to a significant reduction in greenhouse gas emissions, making green gyms an excellent model for sustainable fitness.

Outdoor green gyms, on the other hand, leverage the natural environment for workouts. They are free, open-air spaces with exercise apparatus that encourage cardiovascular workouts, strength training, and muscle toning. They not only feature eco-friendliness through avoidance of energy consumption, but also promote community wellness and interaction by being accessible for all.

3.2. The Environmental Impact of Conventional Gyms

Before we delve deeper into the advantages of green gyms, it's important to examine the environmental impact of conventional gyms. Traditional gym facilities are substantial energy consumers. They operate lights, air conditioning, music systems, and a myriad of exercise machines on a nearly constant basis. Moreover, bottled water and single-use towels in these facilities lead to an enormous waste generation.

A treadmill, for instance, can consume over 700 kilowatts per year when used for five hours each day, equivalent to the power usage of an average household in the US. Similarly, elliptical machines, resistance heaters, and rowers contribute significantly to a gym's overall power demand. With a majority of fitness centers reliant on fossil fuels for electricity, this poses a considerable environmental concern.

3.3. The Green Gym Equipment Revolution

One of the defining features of green gyms is their employment of exercise equipment that generates electricity from workouts. Instead of consuming power, these treadmills, ellipticals, and stationary bikes convert human kinetic energy into sustainable electricity.

A prominently used device in these fitness centers is the SportsArt ECO-POWR line. It includes machines such as the Verde treadmill, the world's first energy-producing treadmill. Powered by users rather than a traditional power outlet, it generates up to 200 watts of electricity per hour of usage. When plugged into an outlet, the power generated goes back to the grid, offsetting the gym's energy consumption, or even contributing surplus energy.

Other brands such as ECO Gym and Green Revolution have also followed suit, providing gym-goers options to contribute towards the 'Green Energy Revolution'.

3.4. Building a Sustainable Atmosphere: Design and Management Approaches

Green gym management extends beyond equipment to incorporate eco-friendly building design, recycling initiatives, and waste management. The design of the gym facilities often includes incorporating green roofs for temperature regulation, deploying solar panels for energy generation, and using recycled rubber flooring and eco-paints.

Water-saving initiatives, such as low-flow toilets and showers, along with automated faucets, significantly reduce water consumption. Moreover, promoting the use of reusable water bottles and providing filtered water taps makes a substantial difference to plastic waste reduction.

Gyms are also transitioning from offering single-use towels to recommending clients bring their own, further reducing water consumption and detergents often used in commercial laundries.

Managing waste effectively also forms the part of green gym management. Providing segregated bins for recycling and composting encourages gym-goers to participate in waste management initiatives.

3.5. Health Benefits: From Improved Air Quality to Active Outdoor Sessions

Switching from conventional to green gyms doesn't just benefit the environment; it contributes significantly to the health of gym-goers as well. Green gyms have highlighted the need and potential for outdoor workouts, and these sessions in natural settings are said to deliver great mental health benefits.

Being amongst nature during these outdoor workouts helps reduce stress, improves mood, and enhances concentration. Gym-goers are reported to feel more revitalized and less tense after training outdoors as compared to indoor workouts.

Moreover, sustainable building materials and better ventilation systems used in green gyms lead to improved indoor air quality, reducing the risk of indoor health issues.

3.6. A Call to Action: Join the Green Gym Movement

The rise of green gyms signals a seismic shift in how we perceive fitness. It proves we can achieve our health and fitness goals while prioritizing sustainability. The green gym movement, though in its early stages, is growing steadily. As fitness enthusiasts continue to become more vigilant about the environmental crisis, and as their understanding improves about how their actions in the gym impacts the bigger picture, it's hoped that this fitness revolution will gain momentum.

Through joining this movement, gym-goers not only reduce their carbon footprint but also contribute to a collective mission for energy production, waste reduction, and responsible consumption. Pledging to a green gym approach takes us one step closer to harmonizing our fitness goals with the health of our planet.

Thus, green gyms represent an inspiring example of how we can adapt to healthier lifestyle choices while making a positive impact on our environment. Our fitness journeys should not only encompass the improvement of our wellbeing but should also serve as a commitment towards the longevity and health of our shared home – planet Earth. This marriage of health and sustainability is the future of fitness, and we must endeavor to make it our present, too. Our actions today will determine both the fitness of our bodies and the health of our Earth tomorrow.

Chapter 4. Embracing Outdoor Fitness: Reconnecting with Nature

The great outdoors awaits as your quintessential workout space. This open gym paints a vivid color palette of vibrancy and energy that can boost both physical and mental health. Structured gymnasiums with their sets of heavy machinery might seem a practical ballpark for fitness enthusiasts. Still, the experience of working out beneath the sky, amidst nature makes for a captivating and refreshing alternative. This chapter will guide you through making the most of the outdoors while imbuing habits that contribute positively to our Earth's health.

4.1. The Benefits of Outdoor Fitness

Outdoor fitness or 'green exercise' as often referred to, encompasses any physical activity that is performed outside, enveloped by nature. This kind of activity can include anything from walking, running, cycling, to more niche exercises such as outdoor yoga or even kayaking. It channels the energy from the exercise, aligning it with nature's serene tranquility, generating added benefits to the practitioner.

Physical benefits are apparent and mostly common to indoor fitness, but the key lies in the fringe benefits associated with outdoor fitness. Working out in nature aids in enhancing mood, reducing depression, anxiety and stress levels, as well as improving self-esteem. Sunlight plays a significant role in providing the much-needed vitamin D, pivotal for bone health, boosting immune system and mood regulation.

In addition to these, being outside can create a sense of connection to the natural world. It's a gentle reminder of our coexistence with nature and its elements, fostering a sense of accountability towards our planet. Outdoor fitness doesn't just make us healthier, it makes us better custodians of the Earth too.

4.2. Adapting Your Workout Routine to The Outdoors

Transitioning to outdoor fitness might feel overwhelming initially. One of the effective ways to transition smoothly is by adapting your existing workout routine for the outdoors. Many exercises that you do inside a gym can be easily replicated outside with minor adjustments and creativity.

Find a local park or outdoor space that suits your convenience and begin with aerobic exercises such as jogging, running, power walking, or cycling — these require no equipment at all. Push-ups, burpees, lunges, and squats can be done anywhere and can make a solid foundation for a strength-building outdoor workout. If you miss your gym bench, find a park bench to perform tricep dips or step-ups. Trees, playground structures, or even the base of a sturdy lamp post can be used for resistance exercises, pull-ups, or inclined push-ups. With the right mindset, the world outside is a gym waiting for you to explore.

Adding flexibility and balance training workouts apart from your regular strength and aerobic sessions can also be quite rejuvenating. Many people find yoga or Tai Chi to be the perfect exercises to perform outdoors because of the special connection one feels with nature during the practice. Activities such as swimming, kayaking, or hiking offer the opportunity to exercise while appreciating nature at its best.

A word of caution: always carry water with you to stay hydrated, wear sunscreen to protect from UV rays, proper shoes to avoid injuries, and follow public rules on the use of outdoor spaces.

4.3. Eco-Friendly Outdoor Equipment

Fitness equipment like weights, resistance bands, yoga mats, etc., made from non-recyclable materials, contribute a significant percentage to global pollution. In promoting outdoor fitness, it's important to consider using eco-friendly outdoor equipment.

Many companies today manufacture fitness products using sustainable materials. For instance, yoga mats made of natural rubber, cork, or jute; weights and kettlebells made of recycled steel or iron; resistance bands made of eco-friendly latex; reusable water bottles made of stainless steel or glass, instead of plastic.

These environmentally conscious choices help reduce your carbon footprint, bringing you one step closer to becoming an Earth-friendly fitness enthusiast. However, the best equipment is your own body. Bodyweight exercises like planks, push-ups or lunges, need no equipment, just your determination.

4.4. Creating a Planet-Friendly Diet Plan

Outdoor fitness is to be complemented with a planet-friendly diet for holistic progress towards our aim. Adopting a plant-based diet or reducing intake of animal products drastically reduces carbon and other greenhouse gas emissions. A diet rich in vegetables, fruits, legumes, seeds and nuts is not only beneficial to your health, but also environmentally sustainable.

Encourage locally sourced, organic produce which uses fewer resources for transportation, reducing carbon emissions. Seasonal foods are usually grown locally and do not need artificial assistance to grow, making them a healthier and eco-friendly choice. Promote waste reduction by planning meals, storing food properly, and composting organic waste.

Drinking plenty of water is another factor not to forget. Always carry a refillable water bottle during your outdoor activities to sustain hydration levels. Drinking the right amount of water promotes cardiovascular health, cools the body, helps cleanse toxins, and contributes towards maintaining a healthy weight.

4.5. Conclusion: A Step Towards Sustainable Fitness

Embracing outdoor fitness is about creating a balance between promoting personal health and upholding responsibility towards Earth. By switching to outdoor activities, your gym becomes as big as your exploration. Add some eco-friendly gear to your collection, paired with an environmentally friendly diet, and you are ready to step into a healthier, greener lifestyle.

As you venture into outdoor fitness, you are not just propelling yourself towards a healthier life, but you're also driving a significant change in the world. In every step you take, every breath of fresh air you inhale during your outdoor workout session, you're making a commitment to your fitness and renewing your pledge to the environment.

With this, we leave you at the threshold of another chapter in your 'Earth-Friendly Fitness' journey. Regardless of what your fitness level is or what form of exercise you prefer, there is room for everyone in the great outdoors. Bask in the sunlight, soak the vitamins, connect with nature, and draw inspiration, for you are not alone; your fitness journey supports the wellness of the planet you share with millions of others.

Chapter 5. Sustainable Fitness Gear: From Fabric to Footprint

In the realm of fitness, the gear we use is as significant as the exercises we perform. The materials that go into production, the manufacturing process, the subsequent footprint they leave, and their disposal - are fundamental aspects that need to be evaluated. Embracing a sustainable lifestyle isn't merely confined to diet and exercise; it extends to the fitness tools we use.

5.1. Understanding the Eco-Impact of Fitness Gear

The environmental impact of fitness gear cannot be neglected. Traditional production methods have considerable negative impacts on the ecosystem. Material sourcing is a significant contributor to the depletion of natural resources, with synthetic materials like polyester and nylon causing harm via their production and disposal. These materials, often preferred for their durability and comfort, are, unfortunately, derivatives of crude oil and release greenhouse gases during production. Further issues arise at the end of their lifecycle - these materials are non-biodegradable, leading to waste accumulation and ecological degradation.

Similarly, manufacturing processes often involve energy-intensive techniques and chemical-laden dyes that pollute water systems when released untreated. Carbon emissions during the transportation of these products, especially when produced overseas, contribute significantly to their carbon footprint.

5.2. Towards Sustainable Materials

The shift towards sustainable fitness gear begins with the materials used in their production. Brands globally are pioneering ways to make fitness gear from recycled materials, botanical resources, and natural fibers like organic cotton, hemp, and bamboo. These natural fibers are renewable, require fewer resources to produce, and are biodegradable.

Organic cotton is produced without synthetic pesticides and fertilizers, reducing soil and water pollution while promoting biodiversity. Similarly, hemp is a sturdy, fast-growing crop that can be converted into a durable fiber. Bamboo, a rapidly renewable resource, is employed to create soft, breathable fabric that is excellent for workout gear.

Recycled materials provide another innovative avenue. PET bottles are transformed into high-quality polyester fiber. Fishing nets and other waste nylon are regenerated into nylon yarn through a process that can be repeated infinitely without degrading the quality, effectively creating a closed-loop system.

5.3. The Role of Conscious Manufacturing

Conscious manufacturing practices are an essential part of sustainable fitness gear. Manufacturers who prioritize reducing energy and water use and minimize waste and emissions during production are the key to a greener future.

Several ways to achieve this include using renewable energy sources like wind and solar power during production, minimizing water use in the manufacturing process, and using non-toxic dyes and finishes. The adherence to fair labor practices also goes hand in hand with sustainable practices.

In terms of production waste, initiatives like zero waste patterns, where clothing designs result in little to no fabric waste, are promising. Additionally, modular designs that allow for easy repair or replacement of parts also extend the life of fitness gear, reducing the need for replacement and therefore consumption.

5.4. Reducing the Carbon Footprint

Fitness gear's entire lifecycle, from production and shipping to use and disposal, should be designed to minimize its carbon footprint. Several approaches help in reducing the environmental weight of fitness gear.

1. Local production: Producing and retailing locally can minimize the carbon emissions associated with long-distance shipping. Local production also contributes to local economies and allows for better monitoring of labor practices.

2. Efficient logistics: Smart logistic planning and consolidating shipping can optimize transportation efficiency, thus reducing the carbon footprint.

3. Low Impact Packaging: The transition to eco-friendly packaging made from recyclable or compostable materials helps in lowering carbon emissions.

5.5. Making the Sustainable Choice

Selecting sustainable fitness gear goes beyond just the product's materials and takes into account the production practices, company ethos, and end-of-life conditions. Here are a few tips to guide your sustainable shopping:

1. Research the brand: Understand their commitment to sustainability. Check if their claims are third-party verified.

2. Consider the product's lifecycle: Look for products designed with

long-term use in mind. Products that can be repaired or recycled
are preferable.

3. Keep an eye on the packaging: Packaging should be minimal,
   made from recycled or recyclable materials, and free of plastic.

By taking factors such as these into account, we can tread more
lightly on the planet, even as we work to keep ourselves fit and
healthy.

5.6. In Conclusion

There's an emerging consciousness in the world of fitness that
recognizes the need for sustainable practice. As we pursue our
fitness journeys, it's clear that the health of the planet is tied to our
own. Despite the complexities, the switch to sustainable fitness gear
is a worthwhile challenge. It encourages a circular economy, brings
business practices into alignment with ecological values, and changes
our relationship with the material world. It all starts with informed
choices, so the next time you're upgrading your fitness gear, consider
their impact, from fabric to footprint. Exciting innovations are
making it ever easier to choose sustainable fitness gear designed to
leave as minimal an environmental impact as possible - a meaningful
stride towards 'Earth-Friendly Fitness'.

Chapter 6. Organic Nutrition: Fuel Your Body Sustainably

The rise in consciousness about environmental friendliness has given birth to a surge of green choices when it comes to the food we consume. With organic farming practices making massive strides, organic nutrition has become more accessible than ever. The benefits it offers extend beyond just personal wellness to environmental preservation.

6.1. Understanding Organic Nutrition

Organic nutrition, simply put, is eating foods that are grown and processed without synthetic pesticides, chemical fertilizers, genetically modified organisms (GMOs), preservatives, or additives. Such foods are also not given antibiotics or growth hormones. This approach seeks to protect and enhance ecosystem health, bolster biodiversity, and promote a balance of nature.

6.2. Health Benefits of Organic Nutrition

The organic nutritional approach is abundant in health benefits. Aside from being more nutritious than conventionally grown counterparts, organic products are free from harmful toxins and antibiotics.

Numerous research studies corroborate the nutritional advantage of organic foods, demonstrating they have a higher number of antioxidants, vitamins, and minerals. Antioxidants, which decrease the risk of chronic diseases like cancer, are estimated to be provided

20-40% more in organic food than in conventional food.

Moreover, consuming organic meats and dairy reduces absorption of dietary antibiotics, reducing antibiotic resistance within your system.

6.3. Picking the Right Foods

Understanding food labels is essential in transitioning to organic nutrition. To ensure food is organic, look for the USDA (United States Department of Agriculture) certified organic label. This certification means the food follows strict organic farming practices.

Alongside, it's wise to build a diet rich in fruits, vegetables, grains, legumes, and lean meats for a holistic organic nutrition approach. While organic junk food may be tempting, remember that it's still junk food. Maintain a healthy diet by focusing on wholesome natural foods.

6.4. Plan Your Meals

Plan your meals around what's in season. Organically grown fruits and vegetables are more flavorful and nutritious. Plus, you're supporting local organic farmers and minimizing carbon footprints during transportation.

Moreover, it reduces waste as seasonal, fresh produce tends to last longer. Planning meals also helps maintain a balanced diet week after week, ensuring you get all necessary nutrients.

6.5. Organic Staples and Super Foods

1. Quinoa: A protein-rich food containing all nine essential amino acids.

2. Chia Seeds: Packed with antioxidants and dietary fibers, they're perfect for your morning smoothie or dessert.

3. Organic grass-fed meat: A rich source of iron, vitamins, and beneficial omega-3 fats.

4. Fresh fruits and vegetables: Always choose organic over conventional where possible to avoid harmful herbicides or pesticides.

5. Organic Dairy: Cheese, milk, or yogurt, which come from cows that are not given antibiotics or hormones.

6. Whole Grains: Foods like brown rice, oatmeal, and whole grain bread.

6.6. Organic Dietary Supplements

Like fitness routines, our dietary needs vary. Depending on lifestyle, overall health, and nutritional needs, some people may need dietary supplements.

When choosing dietary supplements, it's important to ensure they're sourced from organic, non-GMO ingredients. Whether you're supplementing with plant-based protein powders, green superfood blends, or daily vitamins, check for any artificial colors, flavors, or preservatives.

6.7. Budgeting for Organic Nutrition

While organic foods can be more expensive, preparation and smart shopping can make them fit into your budget.

1. Buying in bulk can lead to big savings.

2. Look out for deals at your local farmers market.

3. Grow your produce if you have space.

Remember, the benefits of an organic diet often result in less medical expenses down the road.

6.8. Conclusion

To shift towards an organic nutrition regime, adequate knowledge and consistent efforts are needed. Quantifiable personal health benefits coupled with significant environmental advantages make this a worthy transformation. Partake in this distinctive movement that promises an improved overall health for you and a greener, safer planet for future generations. Remember, when it comes to organic nutrition, you're in it for the long haul, not just for the sake of dieting. Every small step matters, so start today and make a difference.

Chapter 7. Commuter Cycling: Fitness on the Move Towards a Smaller Carbon Footprint

The bicycle stands as a symbol of active and environment-friendly transportation. Many people consider cycling as just a recreational activity or a regular exercise regimen. But taking it beyond that and incorporating it into your daily lifestyle can bring about significant changes. We're talking about commuter cycling here- this is about making cycling a part of your routine, integrating it into your everyday travel to work, to the grocery store, to the gym, anywhere within a reasonable distance. Let's explore more about the benefits it has to offer you and nature.

7.1. The Basics of Commuter Cycling

Commuter cycling is exactly what it sounds like - using a bicycle to commute, instead of a car. Sounds simple, right? Well, it should be! Unfortunately, many cities aren't designed with cycling in mind. However, as awareness for environmental issues grows, so does urban planning for cyclist-friendly infrastructure.

Before you begin commuter cycling, ascertain the viability of your commute. You would find dedicated bicycle paths or lanes in some cities to make your commute safer. In the absence of dedicated tracks, learn about the traffic rules for cyclists in your area and remember always to prioritize safety.

A substantial component of commuter cycling is choosing the right kind of bicycle. There exists a specific 'commuter' bicycle genre designed for this purpose. These have features conducive to everyday commuting, such as a comfortable seating position, baggage carriers, and fenders.

Your bicycle must also be properly maintained for a hassle-free commute. Regular checks on tire pressure, brakes, and gears would help you avoid unforeseen circumstances on your route.

7.2. Physical and Mental Health Rewards

The versatility of cycling, a low-impact workout option, cannot be understated. It suits people of all fitness levels and ages. Cycling utilizes large muscle groups in the legs, aids in muscle toning, improves cardiovascular fitness, and provides strength training. Reports suggest that pedaling to work also reduces the risk of heart diseases by 11%.

Remarkably, incorporating a workout into your commute leads to a happy and productive day. Physical activities in the morning induce endorphin release- the body's natural mood-enhancer. In short, commuter cycling ensures that your journey to work becomes an active, de-stressing workout rather than a stressful slog in traffic.

What's more, exercise before a workday enhances attentiveness, speed, and memory, contributing to workplace efficacy.

7.3. Let's Talk Green

While cycling holds numerous health benefits, it also helps in reducing carbon emissions. A typical car emits about 271 gCO2e/km, whereas cycling emits zero tailpipe emissions. Thus, each kilometer traveled by bicycle instead of a car saves substantial amounts on your carbon footprint.

Further, cycling indirectly reduces household energy consumption. It may seem unrelatable, but by reducing reliance on cars, we decrease the demand for petrol stations and, by extension, the electricity they consume.

7.4. Developing Sustainable Infrastructure

With more urban communities in favor of sustainable living, city planning initiatives across the globe aim at promoting cycling.

The concept of 'bike cities' emphasizes the development of comprehensive & secure bike-lanes & efficient bike-sharing programs. There is a surge in bicycle-friendly infrastructure in urban settings, with an increased emphasis on secure bicycle parking spaces, rent-out schemes, and office facilities favoring cyclist commuters such as shower suites.

In places where distances are substantial, multimodal commuting brings a solution. This approach combines different modes of transport, like coupling cycling with public transportation. For instance, cycling to a nearby bus stop, using the bus for most of the journey, and then cycling again to the final destination.

7.5. Sweating the Odd Stuff Out

Granted, commuter cycling invites some challenges like weather issues or secure bicycle parking. Weatherproof gear works well with colder, rainy climates. Portable lock systems or seeking workplaces with secure bicycle lock-up zones address safety concerns.

To conclude, commuter cycling represents a simple yet significant strategy to intertwining fitness and environmental consciousness. The perks of commuter cycling extend beyond your health and wellness. They go a long way in influencing your surroundings, inspiring others around you, advocating for better sustainable practices, and contributing towards a greener Earth. Take this stride and let your fitness journey be a sustainable one. As the popular saying goes, 'Be the change you wish to see in the world.' With commuter cycling, the change starts with you.

Chapter 8. Mindful Yoga and Meditation: The Untapped Green Fitness Paradigm

Yoga and meditation have been part of human culture for thousands of years, practicing tranquility, balance, and mental clarity alongside physical fitness. Unbeknownst to many, these ancient practices also align with modern sustainability principles, making them an untapped green fitness paradigm. In this chapter, we uncover the inherent environmental benefits of yoga and meditation, giving you tools to anchor your wellness journey in mindfulness and sustainability.

8.1. Why Meditation and Yoga?

Before diving into the specifics of mindful yoga and meditation, it is crucial to understand their significance in the perspective of sustainability. To begin with, both yoga and meditation require minimal equipment. A yoga mat, comfortable clothing, and a quiet space are typically all you need - a sharp contrast to fitness regimes that rely heavily on energy-consuming equipment and expansive facilities.

In addition, these practices foster a deep connection between the mind, body, and the world around us. By cultivating a greater sense of awareness about ourselves and our environment, yoga and meditation can inspire us to live more sustainably.

8.2. Mindful Consumption and Yoga

Our daily consumption patterns play an essential role in our wellbeing and that of our planet. This principle is highlighted in

Patanjali's Yoga Sutras where 'Aparigraha' (non-possessiveness) encourages us to take only what we need – a key to leading a sustainable life.

Mindful yoga can help shift our consumer habits towards sustainability by promoting awareness and appreciation of our material needs. By incorporating mindful yoga into our routines, we can cultivate a lifestyle that embraces minimalism and reduces waste.

8.3. Meditation and Environmental Awareness

Meditation enhances our awareness of the environment by encouraging us to experience the world as it is – not as we think or want it to be. This increased mindfulness can guide us towards a greener lifestyle.

Through regular practice, we begin to notice the subtle but critical role the environment plays in our lives. We become more attuned to the beauty of nature, the consequences of our actions on the environment, and the urgent need for sustainability. This awareness can drive us to make greener choices every day.

8.4. Eco-Friendly Yoga Accessories

Although yoga demands minimal equipment, the market is filled with gear made from non-biodegradable materials. Opting for eco-friendly yoga accessories enhances your green fitness regime. Natural, biodegradable materials like cork and natural rubber are excellent choices for yoga mats. Organic cotton or hemp yoga clothes are great alternatives to synthetic apparel.

8.5. Mindful Yoga Techniques

Let's delve into some yoga techniques oriented towards mindfulness and sustainability. Incorporating these practices into your routine can bring you closer to your green fitness goals.

1. Outdoor Yoga: Practicing yoga outdoors reduces reliance on artificial lighting and air conditioning. Additionally, connecting with nature can deepen your mindfulness practice.

2. Sun Salutations (Surya Namaskar): This series of postures is a great way to start your day. Not only does it energize the body and calm the mind, but it also fosters gratitude for the sun - our primary source of sustainable energy.

3. Tree Pose (Vrikshasana): This balancing pose helps ground us, increasing awareness of our relationship with nature.

4. Aparigraha-Inspired Yoga: This yoga practice focuses on letting go of physical, emotional, and mental clutter. It encourages a sustainable lifestyle via minimalism and mindful consumption.

8.6. Sustainable Meditation Practices

1. Guided Environmental Meditations: These meditations focus on appreciating nature's beauty and understanding our role in preserving it.

2. Walking Meditations: Walking barefoot on grass or sand can enhance grounding and awareness of nature while integrating fitness with a low-carbon footprint activity.

3. Energy Conservation Meditations: These techniques train the mind to observe and control energy usage in daily life. Over time, energy conservation becomes an integral part of your lifestyle.

8.7. Eco-Yoga Retreats

Consider participating in eco-yoga retreats for a full immersion into sustainable living and mindful practices. These retreats teach yoga and meditation with a strong emphasis on sustainability, such as composting, gardening, plant-based diets, and more.

In conclusion, yoga and meditation offer an untapped green fitness paradigm. By promoting mindfulness, minimalism, and reverence for nature, these practices help build a sustainable lifestyle that preserves both personal health and Earth's environment. Incorporating mindful yoga and meditation into your fitness routine can be a transformative step towards a healthier you and a greener planet. Approach each day as a chance to align your actions with your values, blending fitness with sustainability for a holistic wellbeing.

Chapter 9. Green Fitness Trends: The Future is Here!

As we catapult towards an era of heightened environmental consciousness, the fitness industry is not being left behind. This chapter will delve into the latest trends shaping the green fitness movement, grounding its roots in current social and consumer behaviors and casting light into the future of this growing phenomenon.

9.1. From Fast Fitness to Slow Fitness

A new paradigm shift is sweeping across the fitness industry. It is the concept of 'slow fitness.' This approach is about consciously embracing physical activities that are sustainable for both our bodies and our planet. This shift is a departure from the 'fast fitness' culture characterized by high intensity, energy-zapping workouts, and disposable consumerism of fitness gear.

Slow fitness emphasizes undertaking light, regular physical activities such as walking, cycling, or swimming, which are more sustainable for the body over time and reduce the carbon footprint associated with travel to and from gyms. The equipment used aligns with this ethos, advocating for durable, reparability and ultimately reusable products.

9.2. Sustainability Embraced by Fitness Tech

Technology in fitness is progressively embracing environmental consciousness. Startups and big tech companies alike are researching and developing fitness hardware that uses renewable energy sources. The manifestation of this trend is in the form of spin bikes that generate electricity, elliptical machines powered by solar energy, and treadmills that source their power from kinetic energy generated while running.

In addition, fitness technology innovators are exploring eco-friendlier alternatives for tech components such as biodegradable wristbands for fitness trackers and sustainably sourced raw materials for gym machines. The fitness app market is also contributing to this green wave by encouraging at-home workouts, hence cutting down carbon emissions associated with gym commutes.

9.3. Green Gyms - The Ultimate Fitness Spaces

Green gyms epitomize the concept of earth-friendly fitness. These gyms leverage the sustainable design ideas such as efficient energy use, water conservation, and waste reduction. They employ renewable energy systems for power, rainwater harvesting, and reuse systems for water needs, and composting or recycling initiatives for biodegradable waste.

For reducing air travel for international fitness retreats, virtual workouts are streaming high-quality exercise sessions from exotic locations. This is not just eco-friendly but also fosters inclusivity by breaking financial and geographical barriers, allowing more enthusiasts to participate from the comfort of their homes.

9.4. Vegan Fitness - Food Fuelling Fitness

Veganism is making noticeable inroads into the fitness industry. With well-documented studies highlighting the environmental impact of meat and dairy industries, more fitness enthusiasts are turning towards plant-based diets. Vegan fitness pushes for nutrition derived from less resource-intensive food sources like grains, legumes, fruits, and vegetables, as opposed to meat and dairy products.

In addition, there is a sharp increase in the formulation and consumption of vegan protein supplements, debunking the old myth that animal products are the only effective sources of protein for muscle recovery and growth.

9.5. Activewear and Equipment Going Green

As consumers become increasingly eco-conscious, demand for sustainable fitness wear and gear is growing. Brands are responding by developing clothing lines featuring organic cotton, bamboo, and recycled polyester. In addition, initiatives like take-back programs for worn-out clothing items for recycling, and manufacturing fitness equipment from recycled or renewable materials, are gaining prominence.

=== Outdoor Fitness - Nature as Gym

Nature-based workouts are surging in popularity, providing individuals with an opportunity to connect with the environment while keeping fit. Running, yoga, outdoor aerobic classes, and boot camps held in parks or beaches are some examples. Not only does this trend reduce the energy consumption associated with indoor fitness centers, but it also fosters a deeper appreciation for the environment, strengthening our resolve to protect it.

=== Raising Awareness and Encouraging Participation

To ensure the mainstreaming of green fitness trends, awareness and active participation is key. This entails education through various channels about the impact of our fitness choices on the planet and our bodies, and how we can make more sustainable decisions.

Through efforts from us as individuals, fitness industry stakeholders, and everyone in between, we're paving the way for a greener future, where keeping in shape doesn't compromise the planet's health. This era of earth-friendly fitness is not just a fleeting trend but a necessary shift - for our bodies, our planet, and future generations.

Chapter 10. Creating Your Own Sustainable Fitness Routine

Creating a sustainable fitness routine entails more than just constructing a workout plan. It requires integrating habits that respect both your body and the environment. Let's delve into some significant steps on how to establish your own sustainable fitness routine.

10.1. Understand Your Fitness Goals

Before developing any fitness routine, it's critical to understand your fitness objectives. Are you aiming to enhance your cardio, gain muscle, or improve flexibility? Do you wish to lose weight, maintain a healthy lifestyle, or train for a particular sport? Identifying these goals will help in designing a personalized and efficient exercise routine. Always remember to set realistic and attainable goals.

10.2. Design a Well-Balanced Routine

Once your goals are established, the next step is to design a balanced routine. A well-rounded fitness regime incorporates three main elements: aerobic activity, strength training, and flexibility exercises.

1. *Aerobic Activity*: This includes any exercise that increases your heart rate, such as running, biking, swimming, or even walking. Aim for at least 150 minutes of moderate aerobic activity or 75 minutes of vigorous activity per week.

2. *Strength Training*: These exercises focus on building muscle. They

include weightlifting, bodyweight exercises, and resistance band workouts. Aim for 2-3 strength training sessions per week.

3. *Flexibility Exercises*: These exercises, such as yoga, improve the body's flexibility and mobility, enhancing performance in other workouts and preventing injuries. Incorporate them into your routine at least 2-3 times a week.

10.3. Incorporate Sustainable Exercises

The key to eco-friendly fitness lies in the incorporation of sustainable exercises. These include practices that utilize minimal or no equipment and take advantage of natural elements.

- *Bodyweight Training*: This requires no equipment and can be done anywhere. It includes exercises like push-ups, squats, lunges, sit-ups, and burpees.

- *Outdoor Activities*: Choose outdoor activities that have low environmental impacts. Running, yoga in the park, cycling, hiking, swimming in natural bodies of water, and beach volleyball are some excellent options.

- *Green Gyms*: Some gyms have adopted eco-friendly mechanisms like using manually powered treadmills and static bikes capable of transforming kinetic energy to electrical energy.

10.4. Select Eco-Friendly Fitness Gear

Exercise equipment, workout clothes, and even the water bottles you use all contribute to your routine's overall sustainability footprint. Opt for eco-friendly fitness gear where possible.

Exercise Equipment: Look for fitness gear made of sustainable materials. For weights, consider natural fitness gear like sandbags, rocks, or water-filled jugs. If purchasing equipment, opt for those made from recycled or biodegradable materials.

Workout Clothes: Choose activewear made from sustainable fabric such as organic cotton, bamboo, or recycled polyester.

Accessory Choice: Opt for reusable water bottles instead of single-use plastic ones. Use towels made from organic cotton or bamboo fiber.

10.5. Adopt an Organic, Plant-Based Diet

Lastly, your diet is an essential part of your fitness routine. An organic, plant-based diet, rich in fruits, vegetables, whole grains, legumes, and nuts, provides all the essential nutrients. It not only promotes overall health and fuels workouts but also significantly reduces ecological footprint.

10.6. Monitor and Modify Your Routine

Sustainability means adaptability. Your fitness routine should be flexible, adjusting to changes in goals, availability, and even more sustainable exercise options that are continually emerging. Regular monitoring and tweaks keep your regime effective both for your health and the planet.

10.7. Involve Your Community

Encourage others around you to join in your eco-conscious fitness journey. This not only offers a support system and motivation but also multiplies the positive environmental impact.

Recall that the idea is to strike a healthy balance between your fitness goals and sustainable practices. This balance varies from person to person, and that's perfectly alright. Fitness is a personal journey, and every step counts in collective environmental sustainability. Take it one step at a time; remember, every small change contributes to a significant difference.

By implementing these steps, you'll not only foster a fitness routine that benefits your health and wellness, but also aligns with your eco-conscientiousness. As you work towards your goals, you're simultaneously creating a better world for future generations—a world where taking care of yourself and the planet goes hand in hand. Happy, healthy, and green is the new fitness mantra!

Remember, your Earth-friendly fitness journey is an open-ended voyage. It's an ongoing commitment to yourself, your health, and the health of the world around you. Ultimately, it's about creating an eco-conscious way of living, one that redefines the meaning of fitness and wellbeing in the 21st century.

Chapter 11. The Impact of Fitness on Climate Change: A Closer Look

While the connection between fitness and climate change may not seem immediately understandable, they have an intricate relationship that needs careful exploration. This chapter will shed light on how our exercise habits can impact climate change, both positively and negative, and how we can consciously direct our fitness endeavors towards creating a healthier planet.

11.1. The Carbon Footprint of Traditional Exercise

The long-standing practice of using fossil fuels to light, heat, cool, and run machinery in gymnasiums contributes significantly to greenhouse gas emissions. This issue is further exacerbated when we take into account the carbon emissions associated with commute to gyms.

A comprehensive study in 2012 found that the U.S. health clubs consume around 6 billion kilowatt hours of electricity annually. This amounts to three million metric tons of carbon dioxide emitted into the atmosphere each year.

Moreover, manufacturing fitness equipment is not environmentally benign. It involves use of non-renewable resources, production of greenhouse gases during manufacturing, and creation of non-biodegradable waste at the end of the equipment's life cycle.

11.2. The Environmental Aspects of Sportswear and Gear

Another element of the fitness industry with potential negative impacts on the climate is sportswear production. The fashion industry, which includes sportswear, is the second largest consumer of the world's water supply, and emanates about 10% of global carbon emissions – more than all international flights and maritime shipping combined.

Moreover, many athletic shoes and apparel are made from synthetic materials, derived from petroleum. This not only involves extraction of fossil fuels, but also releases carbon dioxide during the manufacturing stage.

Lastly, fabrics such as polyester, nylon, and acrylic can take up to 200 years to decompose in landfills, thereby adding to the pollution.

11.3. Rethinking Physical Exercise for a Greener Planet

Fortunately, there are numerous opportunities for us to reduce our fitness carbon footprint. We can start by taking advantage of the environment around us and engage in outdoor exercises like jogging, cycling, or hiking. These not only provide excellent cardiovascular workouts but also bring us close to nature, deepening our respect for the planet.

Furthermore, bodyweight exercises are a fantastic alternative as they require no specialized equipment. Yoga, pilates, push-ups, squats, and lunges are few examples of such exercises.

11.4. Greening the Gym Experience

While moving outdoor is a great solution, it's understandable that some people prefer the gym environment for their variety of equipment and classes . For those who favor gym workouts, consider using energy-generating fitness equipment. Some companies have developed treadmills, cycles, and ellipticals that produce electricity during workouts.

Choosing gyms that emphasize sustainability in their operation can also make a huge difference. Look for facilities with energy-efficient lighting and machines, alternative energy sources, and a strong recycling program.

11.5. Eco-Friendly Sportswear

The last aspect we'll discuss forms an integral part of our workout routine - the sportswear and gear. Choosing brands that hold strong ecological values can immensely reduce the environmental impact.

Manufacturers are now creating high-performance athletic shoes and clothing from recycled materials and organic cotton. These eco-friendly alternatives drastically cut down on the amount of water and chemicals used during production, thus reducing their environmental footprint.

11.6. The Power of Diet in Your Earth-Friendly Fitness Regime

The final and one of the most significant components of fitness we need to address is diet. Our food choices unimaginably impact our planet's health. By opting for plant-based meals and reducing our intake of meat and dairy, we can significantly reduce the greenhouse gases associated with animal agriculture.

Moreover, choosing organic, locally grown products not only reduces carbon emissions associated with long distance transportation but also supports local economies and avoids harmful pesticides.

11.7. Conclusion

It's evident that our fitness routines can substantially influence climate change. Yet, with conscious and intentional choices, we can ensure these impacts are positive, creating a healthier life for ourselves and a sustainable future for our planet. Incremental changes in our fitness routines can ripple across our globe, promoting a culture of sustainability that goes far beyond the gym walls.

It is our sincere hope that this exploration has brought you a step closer to making informed choices towards an environmentally friendly fitness journey. Remember, every step taken, every weight lifted, and every mile ran can be a contribution towards the planet if made in the right way. Health isn't merely personal; it's planetary.

Remember, fitness is not just a personal endeavor. It's a powerful tool to shape and sustain the world around us. This transformative journey of Earth-Friendly Fitness not only guide you towards personal vitality, it will also instill habits that contribute to the wellbeing of our planet.